30 Things I'd Like You to Know About Bipolar.

Katie Rickson
owner, founder and creative director
of Business in the Bath

Published by Business in the Bath
www.businessinthebath.co.nz

© Katie Rickson 2025

The moral right of the author has been asserted.

Edited by Dawn Adams

Designed and typeset by Imelda Morgan,
Two Sparrows Ltd, www.twosparrows.co.nz

Photo of Katie: Nykie, sheshoots.co.nz

All rights reserved. Without limiting the rights under copyright above, no part of this publication may be reproduced, stored in a retrieval system, or transmitted, in any form or by any means (electronic, mechanical, photocopying, recording or otherwise), without the prior written permission of the copyright owner of this book.

Disclaimer: The material in this book is provided for informational purposes only. The ideas, insights and suggestions contained in this book are not intended as a substitute for consulting with your doctor or other medical professionals. The author and the publisher assume no responsibility for any damages or losses incurred during or as a result of following this information.

ISBN: 978-0-473-75446-4

Contents

Kia ora!... 11

Part One: How I experience the world.

1. Hypergraphia 15
2. Anxiety & panic attacks 16
3. Matter of time................................ 18
4. Hypomania & colour 19
5. Appetite changes............................. 20
6. Insomnia and sleep challenges 21
7. Suicidal thoughts............................. 23

Part Two: Language matters. The different ways people with bipolar can relate to their condition.

8. Manic depression 27
9. Bipolar affective disorder..................... 28
10. Does the word 'disorder' create a divide? 29
11. Bipolar is never a punchline 31
12. Reframing.................................... 32
13. Is it ok to say I AM bipolar?................... 33
14. Self-stigma................................... 35

Part Three: Things that help.

15.	Create	39
16.	Counselling and therapy	40
17.	You're not alone: community	41
18.	Soothe first: integrate later	42
19.	Let yourself be mediocre sometimes	44
20.	The right meds	45
21.	Gratefully grasping at glimmers	46

Part Four: How you can help.

22.	Ask compassionate questions	49
23.	Don't try and fix: offer silence and solidarity instead	51
24.	Community care	52
25.	Support at work	53
26.	Holding space with curious questions	54
27.	Remind them they are loved with mantras, proverbs and affirmations	55

Part Five: Mental health and neurodivergence: The bigger picture.

28. Neurodiversity and neurodivergence 59

29. Mad Pride 60

30. Stories are everything 61

References 64

Want to know more?
Hear me share my story (podcasts) 67

Read more of my writing 67

Book me to speak live 67

Follow me on socials 68

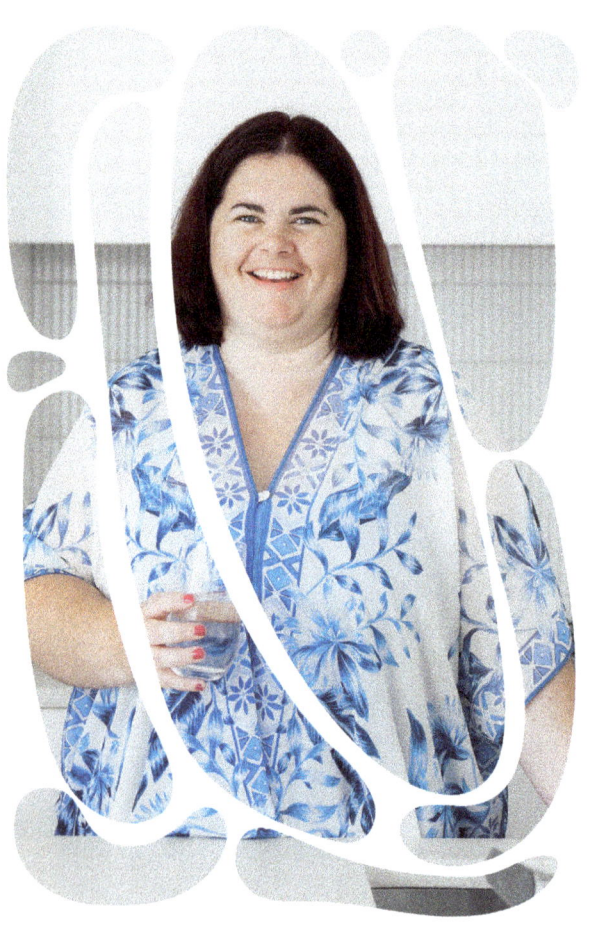

Kia ora!

I'm Katie – a business owner, writer and editor – wife to my amazing hubby, Mike, and mum to our gorgeous 9-year-old daughter.

Nine years ago, when I was freshly postpartum, breastfeeding and adjusting to being a mum, I was experiencing extreme mental distress.

Anxiety, depression, racing thoughts, hypergraphia, insomnia, disturbing breaks from reality, and elevated energy – I was going through it all.

Under the care of Maternal Mental Health, I was formally diagnosed with bipolar type 1.

When you're diagnosed with any long-term condition, it's natural to turn to Google to read what to expect. But sometimes it's scary and not always easy to relate to.

I'd already been living with undiagnosed bipolar for at least 10 years prior to my postpartum episode. I'd already experienced mania, insomnia and hospitalisation.

This means I have lived with bipolar for over 20 years (whether I knew it or accepted it or not). Over time, I've accumulated a lot of lived experience with this condition.

This is the pocketbook I wish I had when I was struggling. Bipolar from a lived experience perspective.

My story is from my perspective, and it's grounded in where I live - the beautiful Aotearoa, New Zealand. I stress that it's "my" perspective of bipolar, and although there will be similarities, everyone's experience is rich and varied. I encourage you to seek out as many different voices and stories of bipolar as you can.

I've written it for people living with bipolar (formally diagnosed or not), their loved ones, decision makers, and those who lead us and support us.

This book is deliberately concise. I originally wrote each topic as a LinkedIn post - so they don't claim to go deep. I hope the different topics pique your interest, and you feel inspired to research further. My mission is for this book to reach the right hands at the right time - and for it to help us live in a kinder, more informed and compassionate world.

I dedicate this book to my family. Thank you to my parents, Helena and Peter, and my in-laws, Daphne and Malcolm, for all your support.

Thank you Mike and Zoe for bringing so much love, hope and fun to my life.

Part One:

How I experience the world

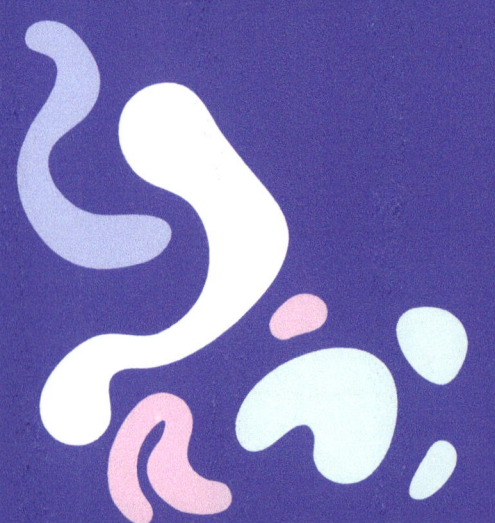

1

Hypergraphia.

I bring pen and paper into the blue tiled tub

That sits solidly

A centre.

I write myself elsewhere.[1]

Hypergraphia forces me to bring pen and paper with me everywhere I go.

It is the intense desire to write (or draw). When I experience this, my writing output increases dramatically.

Flooded with ideas, my writing speeds up. My hand races across the page. My brain - and wrist - 🔥.

Is the writing any good though?

Depends. It's vivid and urgent and raw and an insight into my mind. It usually comes out as a stream of consciousness, or I try and shape it into a poem.

I haven't experienced hypergraphia for a while. I'm not sure if I enjoy it - even though it looks like the opposite of writer's block.

It feels relentless - making it hard for me to sleep and focus on anything else.

2

Anxiety &
panic attacks.

Riley, the main character from *Inside Out* 1 and 2, is sent off the ice hockey rink for foul play. She has a panic attack.

Sweating. Knees shaking. Tears. Heart pain.

The character of anxiety becomes a blur of orange and synapses and electricity. She moves at an unbearable speed – around and around in circles and rumination. Getting nowhere fast, while draining so much energy and hope.

Watching this scene at the movies brought me to tears. I had to hold it together for my daughter and her friend. And no one wants soggy popcorn.

Panic attacks were a regular feature of my life when I was unwell. Anxiety and bipolar often go hand in hand. Whether it's a feeling of being trapped, or unable to see a better future, or insomnia, or regret for something I said or did, anxiety would be there just under the surface. All the time.

That's why I have a lot of compassion for people who live with anxiety and panic attacks.

There is a way through. Some things that help me are being in cold water - a shower, a swimming pool, even holding some ice. People being with me and helping me to slow down my breathing. Having a cry also helps reduce my stress. Guided meditation where you let out a loud sigh for each exhale.

3

Matter of time.

In te reo Māori, the term for bipolar is Mate Rangirua.

Rangirua has several definitions including as a noun: out of tune, out of time, out of sync.

And also as a verb: to be out of tune, out of time, out of sync.

I resonate with the feeling of being out of time and sync. There have been times where I've experienced several hours as if they were 15 minutes. Other times when my circadian rhythm is so out of whack I can't fall asleep. I've experienced time freezing, stretching, condensing.

Losing time too. Feeling stuck in time.

Travelling between time zones can trigger something dangerous.

4

Hypomania & colour.

The vibe is electricity from my sandals to my scalp.

I am standing outside BookMark, a secondhand bookshop stacked with pre-loved tomes and other treasures. I look across the road at the Devonport library. I see the facade and the mature pōhutukawa. The greens look different today. They are pop-de-bob-popping.

So delicious vivid.

Green's not just green, it's malachite. Brown's not just brown, it's cinnamon. Orange? Amber – waiting for something magical to happen.

This is hypomania. When colours are brighter, people are phosphorescent – charged by being exposed to light – life feels sweeter. Music from the cafe feels curated just for me.

Ideas arrive more easily, quickly, loudly, like the London Underground.

This is the time of the global financial crisis before I know what hypomania is.

Now when colours begin to pop, I find myself suspicious. Is this the right level of green? Is this the right tone of red? Am I seeing these colours as I would normally or are they shapeshifting – hinting at something to come?

5

Appetite changes.

I haven't got the stomach for this.

2009/10: depression.

I'm in my early twenties. I normally love my food; I've lost my appetite. Just the other night, I was at an Italian restaurant for a family dinner, and I migrated strands of cheesy, creamy pasta - pasta dripping in Parmesan and bacon - from the west side of my plate to the east. Curling it around and around my fork and abandoning it - untouched, unchewed, unwanted - on the other side.

2016: post-partum mania.

Baby brain has gifted me with an appetite more enormous than usual. I'm waking up to make me and my husband, Mike, a full-English breakfast. With hash browns. And bacon. Beans and toast. On a weekday! And I'm not a morning person! I'm a messy cook; our tiny kitchen bench is uncouth with pans and cracked eggshells and unlined baking trays and Pam's baked bean cans. A few solitary beans - untouched, unchewed, unwanted - congeal at the bottom.

6

Insomnia and sleep challenges.

2009/2010: It's 3am and again I'm pacing the corridors of the Devonport flat I share with two others.

The flat has Victorian features - fireplace, bay window, elaborate ceiling mouldings and sash windows. Normally a fan of that style, it's no comfort to me now.

Unable to sleep. Unable to get any peace. Tormented by thoughts of being a burden and the world would be better without me.

If I do steal some slumber, it's not restorative. I have recurring nightmares. Lucid dreams, which are strange and disturbing. It's like an *Inception* scenario sans Leonardo. I think I've woken from the dream as I'm in my bedroom, only for something else to happen which I know can't be real. A Russian doll of a nightmare within a nightmare within a nightmare.

Sleep is one of the things they tell you is top dog for your mental and physical health. And productivity. And performance. I want sleep that's a blank canvas. I want sleep as an escape. I want sleep as an empty space for eight hours.

But it's yet another thing I can't do. Another thing I'm failing at. Another thing robbing me of any peace.

I want to reassure you; insomnia is not a regular occurrence for me now. I'm in a much healthier space. But I do still get broken sleep and nightmares when I'm stressed. My pills, which I take at night, usually do a decent job of getting me to fall - and stay - asleep. So much so, I'm usually still pretty groggy in the morning.

Any changes to my sleep patterns point to something being off-kilter. Whether I have a reduced desire for sleep or I want nothing but, I need to protect my sleep like it's the prettiest mixed metaphor in the library.

7

Suicidal thoughts.

One of the hardest parts of living with bipolar is the loud, dark thoughts that you don't want to go on anymore. I've been experiencing these thoughts this week and yet I still appreciate and love my life.

Sometimes these thoughts sneak up on me. Sometimes they are loud. They are worse when I haven't slept well and I'm feeling stressed.

It helps to talk about these thoughts with a professional. Talking about it helps alleviate feelings of shame. It is a relief to speak these thoughts out loud and not be judged.

Part Two:

Language matters.

The different ways people with bipolar can relate to their condition.

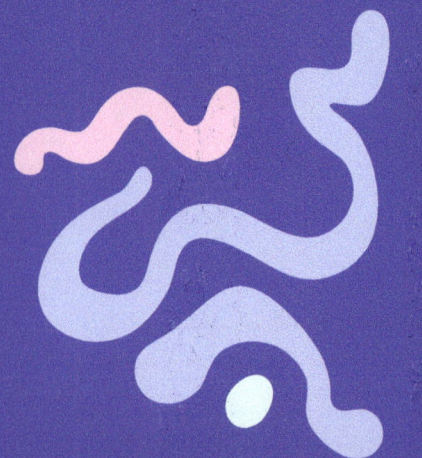

8

Manic depression.

I'm glad they did away with manic depressive as a diagnosis in the 80s. It feels like a reductive way of explaining my experience and that of many others.

To me, it feels heavy, scary and stigmatising. It gives rise to words like maniac and maniacal. Words that are used too flippantly (please can we stop using them in advertising!).

It also doesn't speak to the depth of life with bipolar. It's not just mood and emotional differences – but cognitive and sensory differences too. I don't say deficits or disordered – I'm not a fan of those words either.

There's also more than one type of bipolar which the term manic depressive can't encapsulate.

I found Stephen Fry's film: *Stephen Fry: The Secret Life of the Manic Depressive* very valuable in representing an experience of bipolar. It's interesting, though, that he chose to use the old term – I think when it was made manic depressive was still what most people knew.

It's up to the person living with the condition what they call it, though.

That's the beauty of language – we get to decide which words resonate.

9

Bipolar affective disorder.

Here's another diagnostic term for bipolar: bipolar affective disorder.

Affective in psychology relates to moods, feelings and attitudes.

In psychiatry, it relates to mental health conditions in which mood disturbance, or its expression, is the primary factor.

In other words, bipolar is primarily a mood disorder. More than that, the way we express our moods is disordered.

I'm not a fan of the words "affective" and "disorder" as it relates to my life and experience of bipolar.

It assumes there's a baseline to how we experience moods, feelings and attitudes. It makes me feel like I'm too much, disturbed, disordered. I need to be fixed.

I prefer words like dysregulated, or overwhelmed or emotional differences. States that can be changed.

It brings back a sense of agency and hope. It removes some of the pathologising or othering.

Again, even though we may be diagnosed with a certain name, we get to choose the language we identify with. If it feels heavy or stigmatising, we get to choose an alternative.

10

Does the word 'disorder' create a divide?

The Lived Experience Wānanga - Community Champions Edition, facilitated by Nōku te Ao at the Mental Health Foundation office in November 2023 was brilliant.

In one workshop, we shared words we don't like or avoid. One such word for me: disorder.

Disorder, I think, creates a divide.

This side - the 'Right' - represents people in control of their moods, emotions, behaviours.

The other side - the 'Wrong' side - is disordered, doing life strangely, chaotically, even violently. These disordered people should be subdued, controlled, and returned to the Right side - or so the narrative goes.

No word is perfect. And if we give people the benefit of the doubt, they may be using the word disorder innocently, unaware of the stigma they are potentially perpetuating.

At the same time, if we want progress and compassion, we should never stop listening to people with lived experience. Good intentions do not erase real impact. Language can - and does - evolve all the time.

Condition is less stigmatising.[2]

Please don't take this in a prescriptive or universal sense. I think the best thing is to ask the person living with bipolar how they identify - the language they choose to use to describe their experience. If they prefer bipolar disorder, we shouldn't argue with that!

I opt to simply call it bipolar. It does its job without disorder tagged on the end. What do you think?

11

Bipolar is never a punchline.

I took my daughter to see the live musical, *Shrek* at the Kiri Te Kanawa Theatre in Aotea Square, Auckland. It was a fun show.

But I couldn't get over Princess Fiona singing that a character was "bipolar". I can't remember what it was in reference to, but it was so jarring. Especially when it elicited a laugh from the audience.

Don't use bipolar flippantly, as a putdown or for any other reason than the condition itself. It's a cheap and tired joke.

I'm over the use of the word mania in advertising, too.

You have so many other options.

You're smarter than that.

12

Reframing.

If language matters as much as I've said it does, it's helpful to find other ways to describe your experience of life with bipolar. Words that go beyond the medical model. Words that ring true for you and allow you to integrate this experience into your story.

You don't even need to share your alternative words with others, if you don't want to. You can be poetic and creative. You can borrow from films, plays and novels. You can be inspired by a metaphor or another cultural representation.

The idea is this is for your benefit. You get to choose a reframe, if you want to. It's not about downplaying or romanticising your experience. But for you to have a say in how you choose to relate to it.

I'll go:

- *Sorrow and Bliss* (a stunning book by Meg Mason)
- *Big Mood* (A dark comedy starring Nicola Coughlan and Lydia West)
- Velvet (a word my GP used to describe me – the opposite of Teflon)

What would you add?

13

Is it ok to say
I AM bipolar?

I'm definitely not the first and I won't be the last when I struggle with how I connect my bipolar to my identity.

Do I say:

I have bipolar?

I live with bipolar?

I experience bipolar?

I am diagnosed with bipolar?

I have lived experience of bipolar?

Or:

I AM bipolar?

Sometimes I use these interchangeably depending on my mood and the context.

After I was diagnosed with bipolar, for a while I completely identified with the label. There was no distinction.

Bipolar is Katie. Katie is bipolar. My calendar was built around events like: tests, a brain scan, countless doctor visits for prescriptions, psych appointments, Maternal Mental Health coffee afternoons, staying in respite care, and even time in hospital.

Bipolar became so ingrained in what I did and who I was, I began to believe this was it. Bipolar was the beginning, the middle and the end.

The words "I am" are so powerful. There's a reason why we use "I am" at the start of affirmations.

Maybe it depends on how we feel about the word bipolar. If we find it overwhelmingly negative, then we are more likely to avoid 'I am'. If we are more positive or neutral about it, it feels safer to say 'I am'.

I'm still working this one out. It's a work in progress. It's okay to not have it tied into a neat bow. I don't want to lock myself in a bipolar box; I don't want to carry any shame about it either.

14

Self-stigma.

Struggle	*vs*	suffer?
Service user	*vs*	patient?
Taking medicine	*vs*	compliant?
Thriving	*vs*	absence of symptoms?

Which column - left or right - helps you feel more agency? Which column feels heavy? Which column feels like you're in the driving seat?

Neither column is perfect. But my point is, the language we repeatedly hear or read can be easily internalised.

Self-stigma is real and feels almost inevitable at the beginning. Sometimes its subtle, other times it's in your face.

The language others use - particularly professionals and in the media - can shape our internal monologue for better or worse.

At the end of Part 2, what I most want to achieve is this: for society to be more curious and compassionate about the language we use around bipolar.

Part Three:

Things that help.

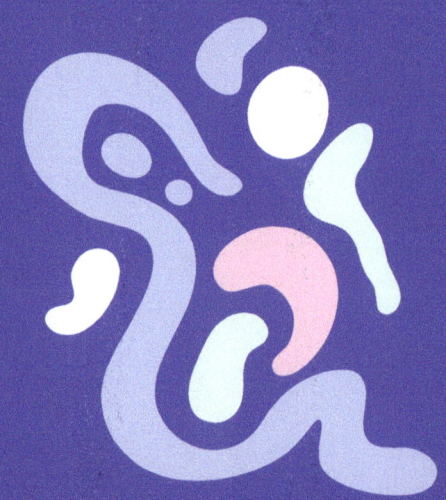

15

Create.

Write through it, paint through it, plant through it, bake through it, improv through it, play guitar through it, draw through it, knit through it, sew through it, dance through it, sculpt through it.

When I want to self-destruct, I create.

There was a reason why so many people turned to sourdough during the pandemic. I never jumped on that trend, but I did bake and draw a lot more than I normally would. I painted rocks and pebbles; hubby created obstacle courses for our four-year-old in the garden.

When we create, we don't even have to be objectively any good. We don't have to be congruent or masterful. We don't have to keep within the lines.

Creating gives us hope and play and agency. Creating together makes community. When we feel like our world – both outside of ourselves and internally – feels so ugly and out of control, creating says there's still beauty to be had.

16

Counselling and therapy.

I see counselling as a rehearsal space. I get to try out different roles and ways of expressing myself. I get to say that hard thing out loud to someone who won't be shocked or offended or run a mile.

I get to see what it's like to speak my truth or set a boundary or talk about subjects which usually make me squirm, without fear of fallout.

And sometimes, I cry. I let myself feel deeply in this safe container. Walking into her space is like entering a Tardis. Those four walls expand to hold every single part of me – the scared 15-year-old who started having recurring nightmares and dark thoughts, the 23-year-old who was taking risks and doing things she didn't recognise, the new mum who had intrusive thoughts, the 38-year-old sharing her story more and more and wondering about the repercussions.

I walk in heavy, and I feel myself shedding skins like a snake.

My thoughts are no longer oppressive; I can be free to explore every part of me. Try it all on for size.*

*This is an excerpt from my upcoming book about creating a life and living with bipolar.

17

You're not alone: community.

You're not alone: three words that can carry as much transformative power as "I love you".

As humans, a lot of us want to be extraordinary at what we do. Extraordinary entrepreneurs, extraordinary academics, extraordinary philanthropists, extraordinary artists.

One thing I don't want to be extraordinary at is bipolar. I don't want to be an outlier. I want community. I want connection. I want to know there are other people like me, seeing life in a similar way to me.

I want representation. I want to see my struggles and triumphs reflected back at me in the media, in books, in positive stories.

18

Soothe first :
integrate later.

I get annoyed when people say baths aren't "proper" self-care.

It's the Western tendency to separate our brains from our bodies, privileging activities that feel cerebral, that feel hard, that stretch us.

But when I feel unsafe and triggered and jump straight to trying to change my mind or behaviour, I feel even more frustrated with myself.

It's like I've skipped a step.

Carolyn Spring, author, trainer, and trauma survivor, wrote in a LinkedIn post:[3]

"The nature of #trauma means that we need to first and foremost calm and soothe our neurobiological state, rather than just trying to change our mind or behaviour. Calm before convince!"

Only when we feel safe, grounded and actually in our bodies, can we do the harder stuff.

So, like most things, it's not either/or. It's not: either have a bath or make that hard phone call; either go for a walk with a friend or leave a toxic environment; either do something that feels good or step outside your comfort zone.

It's AND/AND.

I love how Carolyn writes "re-regulation must always precede integration."

There are lots of techniques for regulating ourselves in times of emotional and sensory distress. Sensory modulation is one way – using your senses to soothe or energise you.

Also, you can't go wrong by checking out *The Neurodivergent Friendly Workbook of DBT Skills* by Sonny J Wise.[4]

19

Let yourself be mediocre sometimes.

Not everything has to be a mic drop moment. Not every post needs a massive response. Not everything needs to be brilliant.

You see, if you struggle with depression, like me, those seemingly mediocre acts of getting out of bed, brushing your teeth, leaving the house are marvellous. When your thoughts seem against you, having a bath, making a cup of tea can be the bravest thing you do.

Not every day needs to be optimised, fine tuned, your best self on show.

We don't have to strive all the time. Mediocre can be marvellous.

You're still here. You're still loved. You're still enough.

20

The right meds.

It's not the whole picture. But I'd be wrong in talking about things that help me without mentioning my meds.

Medication isn't without its side effects. And it isn't for everyone. I believe in medical autonomy and the right to informed choice.

It's a legitimate worry that medication can sedate you too much, can tranquilise you too much and smooth out every emotion - including the emotions you might want to feel more of, like joy. This could be down to the type of medication, the dosage, and when you take it. I'm not a doctor or psychiatrist, so I can't give you advice - all I can do is speak from experience. I take my medication at night, and it helps me sleep. I still have some effects - it takes me a while to warm up in the morning - but I've found ways to tolerate and adjust my expectations of what I can achieve first thing.

Sometimes it can take months, if not years, to find the right medication at the right dose. Some medication - like antidepressants - might potentially lead to a hypomanic or manic episode. That's why it's so important you get the right diagnosis and speak to the right professional.[5]

For me, medication allows me to make the changes to my lifestyle. It gives me a leg up so I can do the harder things. It's not a crutch or a weakness; neither is it the entire picture.

21

Gratefully grasping at glimmers.

Glimmers: feelings of joy and safety and peace.

I wanna make a point of noticing these: the kingfisher that lands on a zip-line, a handwritten card from a friend, a new flavour of chocolate, watching *Derry Girls*, picking up that book from the library you put on hold six months ago because it's finally arrived.

Watching the moon rise over the hills, beautiful prose that defrosts you, a kind message from a new connection, singing together, ocean swims, surprising LinkedIn posts, memes from friends like pebbles from penguins, buttery croissants, *Britain's Got Talent*'s golden buzzers.

When people ask, 'how are you?' more than once - they can tell your first answer is not the whole truth. You end up at their place for a chat and a cry and a cup of strong tea with one sugar.

The way your cats curl up their body and paws just so, getting into a flow state, sharing in anything silly your kid suggests (like playing Granny's Green Underpants – Google it).

Alliteration. Autonomy. Awe.

Part Four:

How you can help.

22

Ask compassionate questions.

"Why?" is meant to be a magical question. "Know your why", "five whys" and all that. And I get it - knowing what motivates us is crucial.

But there's a time and a place.

Why are you depressed?

Eeek. Depending on who asks you this it can fill you with dread and shame. Is there a reason? Is there one reason? How do I even begin to articulate this? Do I even meet the criteria to be depressed?

You are walking on existential ice with far reaching cracks.

I'd say try and steer clear of this question, especially if someone has just opened up to you about what they are experiencing.

More helpful questions could be: Can you tell me what's going on for you right now? What do you need? How can I help?

So, while "why" is powerful in the business world, it can feel intense, and shame ridden when you're speaking to someone about their emotional distress.

I think doctors and other professionals should not initiate a discussion with a why question like "Why are you here?" But instead, a softer "What can I do for you today?" or "What brings you here today?"

Why places the onus on the individual and can make them feel defensive.

What and how feels like an extended arm and a willingness to build a relationship.

23

Don't try and fix: offer silence and solidarity instead.

Sometimes it's too hard to talk. Sometimes asking questions is inappropriate. Sometimes silence and solidarity are the most healing thing you can offer.

15 years ago (how can it be that long?) when I was really unwell for an extended period of time, a friend invited me to her place.

She let me spend the whole day on her couch. She put a blanket over me and her cat made himself at home on my lap.

We might have had the TV on in the background. I know she brought me tea and biccies. I felt so loved and looked after that day.

When you are supporting a friend through mental health challenges, you don't have to have the answers. You don't even have to have the questions. But if you have the time, your friend will remember it always.

24

Community care.

We need to have the systems, support and scaffolding if we are to thrive. The onus isn't purely on the individual, as a society there's lots we can do to help people with bipolar (and by extension other forms of neurodivergence).

Something I really benefited from was respite care which I accessed postpartum under the care of Maternal Mental Health.

Respite care is fantastic because you are still in the community, in a familiar, home-like environment. You have kind and qualified support helping you round-the-clock. They helped me with my daughter so I could catch up on sleep. They did some of the night feeds, or night changes when my daughter was little and they had occupational therapists on hand. Respite care is a dignified way of providing support, it's taking you away from the stresses of life – they cook for you, you have beautiful peaceful bedrooms and it's in a nice setting.

I'm really grateful I was able to access respite care when I was unwell. It points to the social model of health – when we feel cared for, when we have nutritious meals, when we don't feel like we're separated like we might be in a hospital ward.

Respite care was a vital part of my recovery – our policymakers and decision-makers need to value it, invest in it, and make it as accessible as possible.

25

Support at work.

How can leaders step up if an employee discloses they have bipolar?

The top thing for me is flexibility. Flexible start times. Flexibility to work from home if needed.

Flexible targets: for example, spreading deliverables across a month or a quarter rather than expecting the same output every week.

And, just as importantly, a flexible mindset. Today's leaders need to be prepared to have their minds changed about what's possible with bipolar. Don't assume. Stay curious and compassionate. Don't make decisions without us. Make it easy for people to ask for and be granted accommodations.

Many CEOs and senior executives live with bipolar. So much so, that it's often called the 'CEO's disease'.[6] Now, I'm not a fan of the word disease, but it goes to show that living with bipolar doesn't mean you have to give up your ambitions, passions and interests.

But you do need to take flexibility seriously.

26

Holding space with curious questions.

Why are you like this? Why did you react that way?

Sometimes we are genuinely concerned when someone behaves a certain way. Bipolar can feel like a lot to witness and hold space for.

But I want to try and encourage you to avoid the "why" question. It can come across as an attack. I've found there's a lot of power in these phrases instead:

"I'm curious about…

"Can you tell me more about…

"I don't understand. But I want to. Can we talk?"

Sure, there's more words – but these come from a place of curiosity and compassion. They don't feel like an interrogation, but love.

27

Remind them they are loved with mantras, proverbs and affirmations.

Lyrics, proverbs, whakataukī, mantras and even single words can be so comforting to meditate on in times of distress. Like people, they seem to find us at the right time – a serendipity of sorts.

We can be scared that their (over) familiarity empties them of their impact.

But when memory becomes flimsy, the familiar and easily memorable can be a balm. When your brain is yelling cruelty, and all around you seems chaotic and urgent and awful, you can carve out a corner of truth and beauty.

Here are some of my favourite phrases and words to meditate on:

Something beautiful will come from this

I'm at peace with my pace

He tangata, he tangata, he tangata

Manaakitanga

Do you know if your loved ones meditate on any words or mantras? Can you ask them?

Maybe you could leave a surprise handwritten note in their lunchbox or on the fridge so they can see it when they wake up.

Part Five:

Mental health and neurodivergence:

The bigger picture.

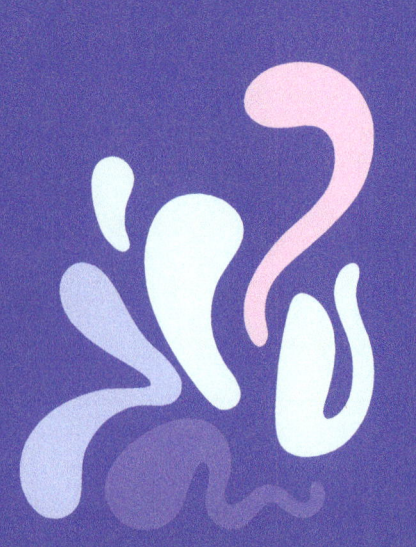

28

Neurodiversity and neurodivergence.

When I was invited to speak at a MUV Talks event on neurodiversity, my first feeling was pride. Quickly followed by: *I'm an imposter.*

I had a narrow idea of neurodivergence. I thought it was for people with ADHD, autism, dyslexia, dyspraxia, and similar. Not bipolar or other mental health conditions.

That you had to be born with it to identify as neurodivergent.

I was wrong.

"People with mental health conditions get to identify as neurodivergent too." Sonny J Wise

I love the advocacy and education work of Sonny J Wise in this space.

Neurodivergent is a socio-political term that's inclusive, expansive and affirming. It doesn't see people's differences as deficits. I can get behind that!

I recommend giving Sonny J Wise a follow and taking a look at their work. It will certainly open your mind - and heart - to a different way of viewing mental health.

29

Mad Pride.

There's another movement I want to tell you about: Mad Pride.

Have you come across it?

I first came across the term at a symposium in 2017. It's about reclaiming the word "mad". Reclaiming the narrative of what it means to live with mental health challenges, to be proud of what we've survived, and to reduce the stigma associated with mental health.

It shares a lot of similarities with the neurodiversity movement in that it's part of your socio-political identity. It's about stepping out of feelings of shame and into a life of autonomy and self-determination and, well, pride. Pride for a life where we feel like we can embrace who we are and fully participate in our recovery.

Of course, it's also about being part of a global community and realising you're not alone.

I was diagnosed with bipolar almost nine years ago. With each year, I feel like I'm shedding the shame, stigma and shadows and fully embracing what bipolar means to me.

30

Stories are everything.

I'm closing this pocketbook with a chat about labels.

Labels can put you in a box if you let them. Labels can stop you from pursuing opportunities. Without visibility and without talking about labels, you can face more self-stigma and stigma from others.

But labels allow you to make sense of your experience, too. Labels allow you to show compassion for some of the behaviours and thoughts you struggle with.

Labels open up access to new understanding of communities like the service user community, the neurodiverse community, and the Mad Pride community. Labels help you access the right support and regain a sense of control and agency.

Labels allow you to take your experience seriously. There's a reason why you're behaving, feeling, thinking, and sensing the world this way. It's not your fault. Neither should you be ashamed of it.

I was diagnosed with bipolar in 2016. It took me a while to get my head around this. This word. This new label. This new lifelong label.

For a while, I completely identified with the label. There was no distinction. It was me, myself and bipolar.

But things have changed during my recovery. One of the most important things for me is to accept that label, make it work for me, and even learn to thrive with that label.

And one of the biggest, BIGGEST things in my recovery has been to seek out other voices, other people living with bipolar – reading and listening and absorbing the different insights on how to live a rich and fulfilling life with bipolar.

I've said it before, and I'll say it again: we must never underestimate the power of stories.

What's my story taught me?

I've realised self-employment works for me, that mental health days are not a luxury but a necessity. It's made me realise bipolar can be the worst at times, but it comes with strengths like creativity, writing, and holding space for other people.

It's made me realise that people and community are everything. It's made me realise I'm resilient. I can bounce back and make sense of the hard experiences.

It's made me realise society has to step up. Society's sicknesses – greed, cruelty, violence, misogyny... the list goes on – need to be addressed if we are all to feel better and more connected with ourselves and each other.

With visibility comes vulnerability and emotional labour. And not everyone can afford to be visible or vulnerable. It's made me realise we all have different relationships with our labels. And that's totally ok.

Like anything in life, recovery requires a village. It's impossible to go it alone. Recovery's a collective slog and a collective triumph. I let my husband in on how I'm feeling rather than trying to carry on and hold it in. Bit by bit, month by month, I've told more people about my diagnosis.

If you live with bipolar, you get to decide your comfort levels around sharing your condition with others. It's totally your call *how* you share it, *when* you share it, *where* you share it, and *who* you share it with. Go slowly, check in with yourself regularly and how it feels, and you can always practise with a trusted professional first.

References

1. Excerpt of my poem, "Expecting". Also published in *The Poetical Lobe. A Community Poetry Anthology*. Vol 1. Edited by Dr Loredana Podolska-Kint. Shared with permission.

2. See this article for more on why 'condition' is a less stigmatising word: www.psychologytoday.com/us/blog/the-i-m-approach/202102/we-perpetuate-stigma-when-we-label-people-as-disordered

3. Read more about Carolyn Spring and her work here: www.carolynspring.com

4. *The Neurodivergent Friendly Workbook of DBT Skills* by Sonny J Wise. Available to purchase: www.livedexperienceeducator.com/store

5. From /ibpf.org/learn/education/treatment/

    "Be extremely cautious with antidepressants...they can trigger mania or cause rapid cycling between depression and mania in people with bipolar disorder."

6. See this article for more info: https://hbr.org/2024/06/3-ways-to-support-employees-with-bipolar-disorder

Want to know more?

Hear me share my story (podcasts).

https://linktr.ee/compassion.poetry

Read

more of my writing.

I share my poetry and writing on bipolar, recovery, motherhood and more here:
www.compassionpoetry.co.nz

If what I share resonates, please become a free or paid subscriber to my Substack:
https://katierickson.substack.com/

Book me

to speak live.

Book me to speak at your organisation:
www.businessinthebath.co.nz

Invite me to feature on your podcast:
katie@katierickson.co.nz

Ask me to deliver a keynote at your symposium or conference.

Follow me

on socials.

Follow me on LinkedIn:
www.linkedin.com/in/katie-rickson-writer/

Instagram:
@businessinthebath

www.ingramcontent.com/pod-product-compliance
Lightning Source LLC
Chambersburg PA
CBHW06205529042 6
44109CB00027B/2829